STRESS SOLUTIONS

PROVEN METHODS ON HOW TO LIVE WITHOUT WORRY

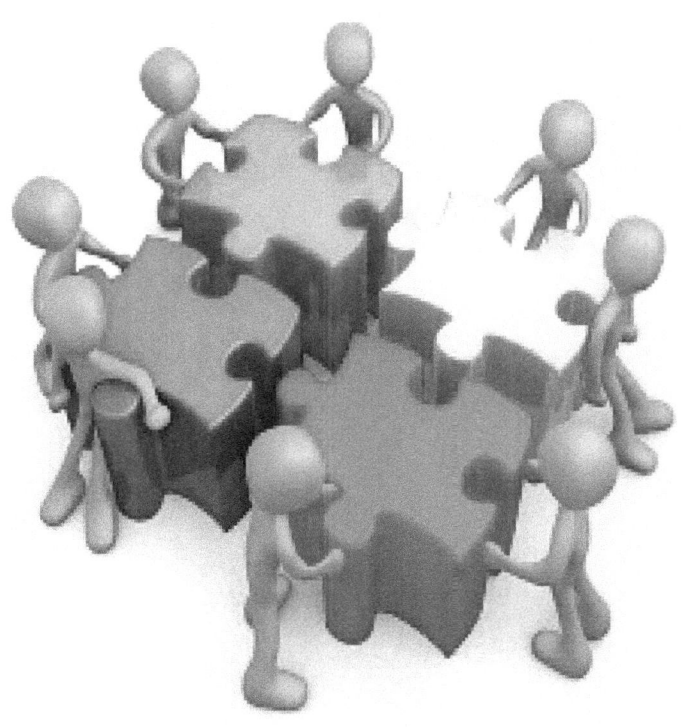

By Patricia A. Carlisle

Introduction

I want to thank you and congratulate you for choosing the book, *"**STRESS SOLUTIONS: Proven methods on how to live without worry**"*.

This book contains proven steps and strategies on how to live without worry.

Worries are something that each and every person experience every day. But not everyone experiences worrying in the same manner or even to the same degree. Everyone has unique sources of worrying of their own. So why are some people so worried about something that's uncertain in the future whereas others merely worry about something after it happens? Let's find out why.

Thanks again for choosing this book, I hope you enjoy it!

TABLE OF CONTENT

Chapter 1

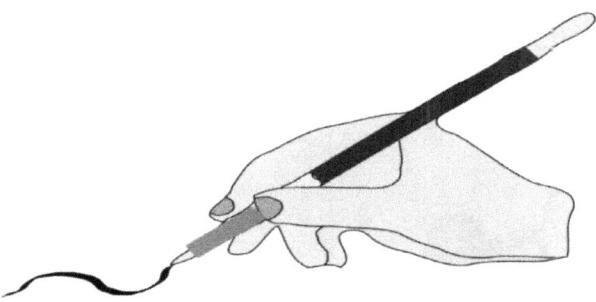

WRITE YOUR WORRIES DOWN

Writing down all of your anxiety and problems before an important exam may facilitate decreasing of test-taking worry, in line with a 2011 study in Science.

Although exams aren't any longer a serious problem to most of the people, an associate professor in psychology at the University of Chicago stated that this approach may work for individuals facing anxieties about different things.

Moreover writing down your worries allow you to let go the burden of keeping track of your problems in your mind. It will be easier to just write them down and review and think about the solutions for your worries in a designated period of time rather than trying to keep record of all your worries in your mind.

Chapter 2

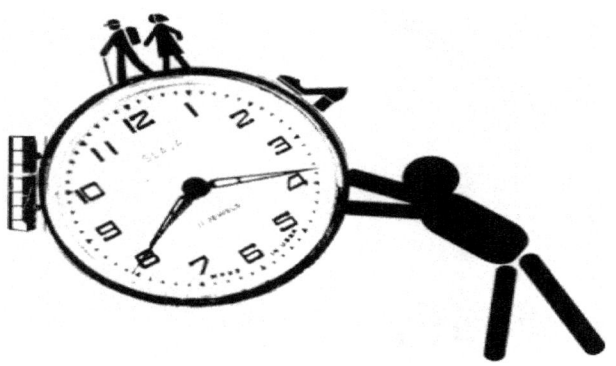

SET ASIDE A DESIGNATED "WORRY TIME"

During A 2011 study, Penn State researchers found that a four-step worry management procedure may facilitate seriously stressed individuals take charge of their anxieties.

Step 1: Determine the cause of worry.

Step 2: Schedule a time and place to accept aforementioned worry.

Step 3: If you notice yourself worrying at a time apart from your scheduled time you need to make yourself think about something else, probably something that calms you down. You could also try and engage in some work that would calm you down.

Step 4: Use the scheduled time economically by thinking of solutions to the causes of your anxiety. So instead of worrying all day, everyday designate a thirty minute amount of your time where you'll be able to ponder about your issues and come up with solutions.

Chapter 3

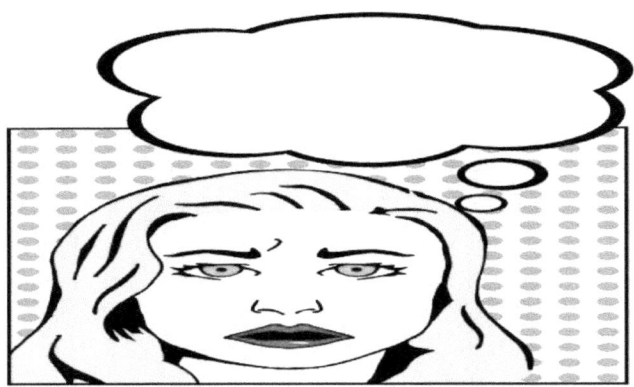

CUT YOURSELF SOME SLACK

Dr. Susan M. Love, a professor at the David Geffen School of medicine at the University of California, at Los Angeles stated to the New York Times that the perceived need to follow all the medical concepts that involves health is a main source of stress and worry.

It's not possible to possess excellent health, and you are most likely lots healthier than you realize. It's never a good idea to consult the internet whenever some small symptom appears that concerns you. A lot of people tend to unnecessarily worry about their health after consulting the internet on such occasions. If you're worried about a symptom you should discuss it with a qualified doctor and understand the real reasons behind it, which is probably nothing most of the time.

No one is able to live forever the aim is to live as long as you'll be able to with the best quality of life you can achieve. Thus, it is of paramount importance that you do not unnecessarily worry about your health, which is ironically not healthy for you.

Chapter 4

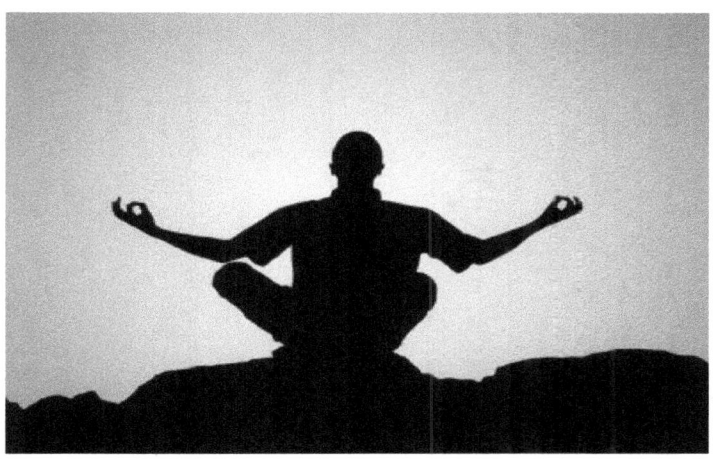

MAKE TIME FOR MEDITATION

Meditation is relatively new but an effective method that has been recognized by a lot of psychologists and psychiatrists. A study published earlier this year in the journal Social cognitive and Affective Neuroscience proved that meditation helps to lower the stress levels in people.

Furthermore it had positive effects on the anterior cingulated cortex which controls the emotions and ventromedial prefrontal cortex, which controls the "worrying". Taking your time to seek out some effective methods of meditation will surely aid in the process of taking control of your worries and leading a happy content life.

The most common and effective method of meditation devised by a lot of psychologists is known as "Anapanasathi" meditation. It basically stresses on the relaxing of your mind by strictly concentrating only on the process of breathing in and out.

Chapter 5

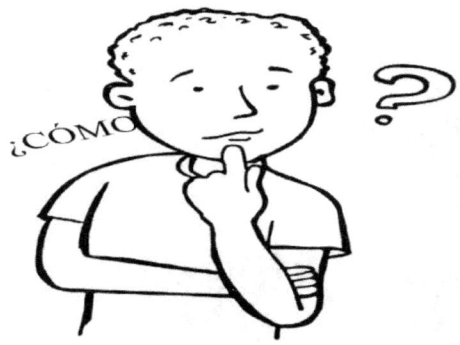

ACCEPT THE WORRY

A 2005 study in the journal Behavior Research and Therapy showed that people who naturally try to suppress their unwanted thoughts tend to get more stressed by aforementioned thoughts. And people who are naturally more accepting of their worries are less troubled, lower in level of depression, and are less anxious, were the conclusions of researches conducted by the University of Wisconsin-Milwaukee researchers.

Worrying about worrying is a dangerous vicious cycle to fall into. Therefore one should try to accept their worries and avoid trying to suppress those. Suppressed thoughts naturally tend to rise up like a rubber ball that's held forcefully under water. Unexpectedly, the suppressed worries might surface causing even worse problems than those of when you're trying to accept them.

Chapter 6

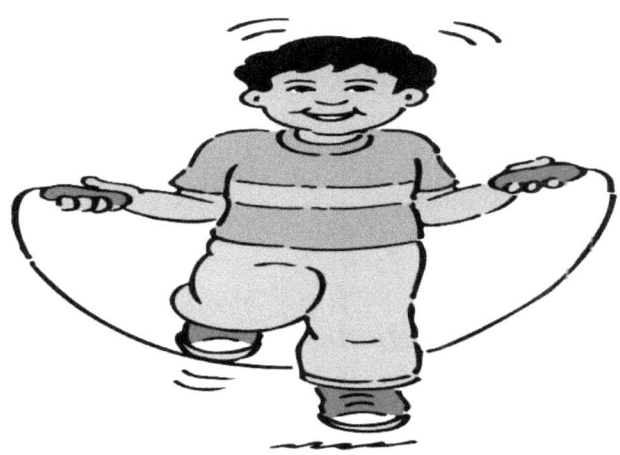

GO OUTSIDE, WORK OUT

The New York Times reported that studies conducted with animals, shows that exercise will have an effect on brain activity of serotonin (an alleged "happy" brain chemical) and also cut back the negative effects of oxidative stress.

Although exercises are said to reduce the stress levels of people, it is important to pick the right kind of exercise schedule for you. For instance a heavier exercising schedule for a person who just took up exercising would cause in inability for him to keep up with the schedule and that would become a source of stress for him.

Moreover, exercising need to be done regularly and consistently, in order to have a considerable positive impact on your mental health. And Well Good stated studies showing that exercise interventions may result in lower anxiety levels that people that keep tied to the couch.

Aerobic exercises are another proved way of dealing with worry and anxiety. Anxiety always pairs up with adrenaline during periods of worry and anxiety and your body is filled with adrenaline. Using that excess adrenaline for aerobic activity can be an effective method to cut back your anxiety and worries. Listed below are few of the myriad advantages of aerobic exercised to relieve from your worries and controlling your anxiety.

- *BURNING AWAY THE STRESS HORMONES.*

- *RELEASING OF ENDORPHINS WHICH WOULD HELP IN IMPROVING YOUR OVERALL MOOD.*

- *EXERCISE IS A HEALTHY DISTRACTION.*

Very basic aerobic activities, for instance light jogging or even fast walking, can be extremely effective at relieving you of you worries, as well as your anxiety itself.

Chapter 7

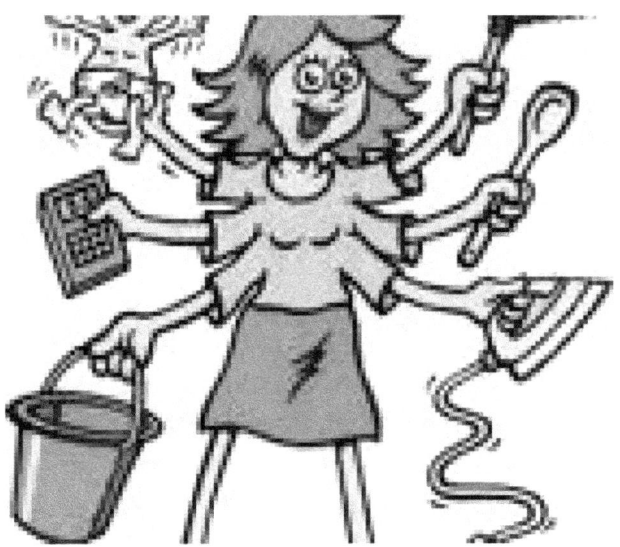

KEEP YOURSELF BUSY

Engaging in activities that keep your hands busy and mind distracted could help prevent flashbacks from traumatic experiences, according to research from the Medical Research Council in England. Although the study didn't include about the validity of the above concept on everyday stress, engaging in activities that keep your mind concentrated may aid in the ceasing of constant reminders of your worries.

After you find a set of things that would calm you down the next important step is to make sure that you put them into action. May be you want to try something that you haven't tried before. But postponing whatever you have in mind due to some reason would be lead into even more stress and worries. Thus it's advised that you put into action whatever you had in mind as soon as possible. Whether it's a bath, a shower, playing outside, getting a massage-if it works for you, do it as soon as possible, rather than let yourself become overwhelmed by your worries further.

When it comes to keeping your mind concentrated on one thing music is good way of doing that. Music, not surprisingly, is a very goodtime tested way of dealing with worrying. Every little thing matters, even if 'it's listening to your favorite kind of music it will have a powerful positive effect on your worrying. As much as it's important to pick your favorite kind of music it's important to not choose loud and noisy music because they naturally tend to release hormones associated with anger and stress. The key is also to make sure you're listening to music that represents the way you want to feel. To some extent, make sure it's calm and slow relaxing music, don't just pick music randomly.

Some might think there's no truth behind the fact that sex is a way of coping with worrying. Sexual intercourse can be incredibly calming. It is a distracting physical activity that releases endorphins and helps you feel more relaxed instantly.

If you have someone special in your life that understands that you're suffering from anxiety and is willing to share in some lovemaking in order to help you experience some relief from the worries, the two of you can come to some type of understanding that allows you to release some sexual energy, and possibly improve your relationship in the process greatly.

Chapter 8

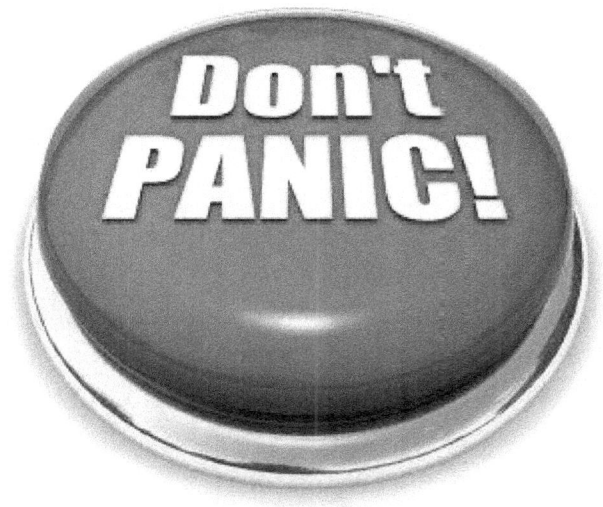

ELIMINATE "WORRY TRIGGERS" IN YOUR LIFE

Cognitive-behavioral therapist has confirmed that we can actually train our brains to respond differently to events. They have partitioned the process of worrying into three basic parts. Namely they are Triggering event, irrational belief and resulting emotion. The process of a person getting worried about a problem is explained as follows.

If someone has an irrational belief about some issue, a triggering event can cause the person to worry about the aforementioned issue. So when something happens that triggers worry, you need to spend some time thinking about what's the irrational belief that's' making you worry and try to see the issue in hand in a different more pragmatic and rational angle.

As mentioned, in theory, looking at your worries in is the key to free yourself from your worries, but how practical is it? You might not always be able to do that on your own. The help of another person, someone close to you is essential in the process of overcoming your worries. If you're tired of your negative feelings like worry and anxiety bossing you around, recruit some help along this process.

Choose someone close in your life to be your motivator reminder. They can remind and motivate you to be rational when you're not. Psychology Today stated, "You have to decide to be the one in charge of your emotions, or your emotions will take charge of you." Use this person to help you talk through your emotions and identify the thoughts that are simply not rational. As mentioned before we can train our brains to react differently to situations. With this process of identifying the irrational thoughts behind your worries you can train your brain to not react with worry whenever a problem occurs; but to reach the problem with a more practical angel and find a solution without worry burdening you down.

Worries and anxiety are not rootless. There is always a triggering action behind every period of worrying you go through in day to day life. Involuntarily your mind can lead you down a path of worries due to triggering events that you don't even notice. Sometimes you can control these worries by being aware of what your triggering actions of worrying are, and keeping those thoughts or events at bay. The more you master at controlling and staying away from those triggering actions the less worried you'll be.

For many, this is easier said than done. But there are many different strategies you can try that may be effective. The first and the most basic step are to eliminate out one of the most common reasons of irrational worrying among people. Most of us tend to worry about a lot of things without any real evidence or facts that clearly shows something is wrong. The cause of worrying here is not being rational and not being aware. So whenever you feel worried you should first question yourself with the two questions mention below.

1. What evidence is there that something is wrong?

2. Is there a chance I'm blowing this out of proportion?

As elaborated above the mind can make you feel worried even for the slightest things, involuntarily. Therefore whenever you feel worried or stress take time to think about the root cause for your worrying, and not it down. Make a list. If possible try and think of ways to avoid the items in your list and put them to action whenever you can. Prevention is always better than cure.

Chapter 9

CONTROLL YOUR ON-LINE ADDICTION

A study from Anxiety United Kingdom showed that just about fifty percent of individuals feel "worried or uncomfortable" being aloof from email or Face book. Seems like all that time you stay staring at your Face book newsfeed, most likely is not doing your psychological state any favor.

It was concluded that most individuals are in serious need of quality time away from their email and social media. Moreover, they stated that people need to reestablish their control over email and social media rather than letting those control one's life. Start with spending a portion of you free time away from your phone and computer, and concentrate on something else that you're interested in.

Chapter 10

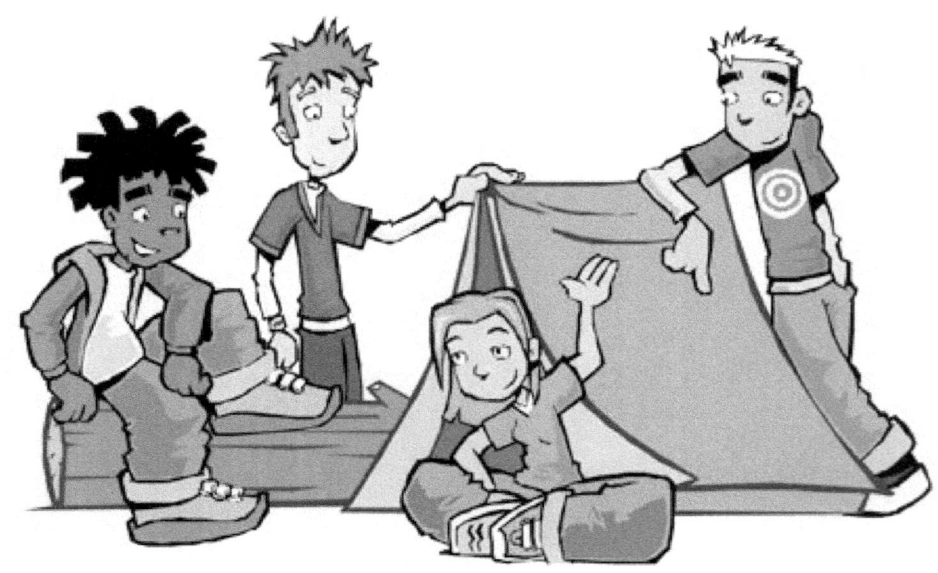

LIVE IN THE PRESENT

A common characteristic of every kind of worrying is that you are worrying about the future. You're scared that something might not turn out like you want it to be or you're worried that something might go wrong that will adversely affect your life. Focusing too much on what's in the store for you is the root of worrying.

Thus an effective way of coping with worries is simply living in the present. Focus on everything that you're interacting with right now. Your duties and obligations and the people you love, everything that you do for fun. Stop worrying about the future do everything you can do to make the future the way you want it, but have no regrets if something doesn't work out the way you want.

Those with anxiety often start to focus too much on how they feel and their worries about the future. Don't make each day a battle against your worries, live with the hope that tomorrows going to be better and work hard for it. Learning that every person is dealing with worries each and every day and deciding to live a happy exciting life anyway is important.

And what's interesting is that if you can learn to finally have that mindset, to let yourself experience worries and decide to live the life anyway and work hard for it worries will affect your life lesser than they did yesterday.

Chapter 11

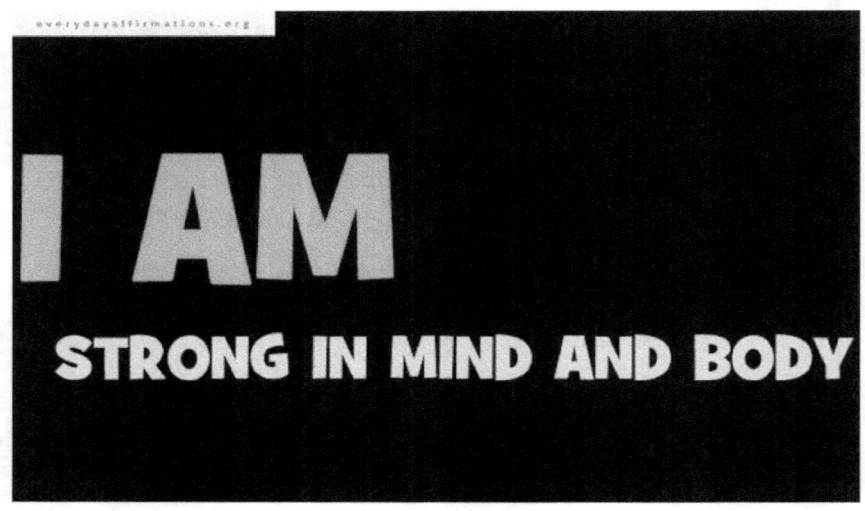

AFFIRMATIONS

Another way to control your anxiety is affirmations. Some people find this way of coping with worries very beneficial. Affirmations are things that you say to yourself to make yourself feel better. For instance consider the example below.

"I'm okay. This is just temporary and I will get over it."

"This is just one drawback I'm looking forward to tomorrow."

Finally, apart from all the adverse effects of worrying and apart from all the ways to control worrying, worrying is a natural mechanism humans have gained to be alert and plan about how something should be done without causing a problem.

Sometimes worrying is necessity. For example if you're in a jungle and you run into a tiger you ought to be worried because unless you're worried about your life and take steps to prevent any damages to your life from the tiger, the tiger will harm you. Therefore necessary worry is something built in to protect you from real dangers.

Content in the above paragraph lead us to the question "Then how much should I worry?" It's not possible to measure the degree to which you should be worried about things, with a numerical value. It depends on the person. Generally, if worrying about something interferes with your day to day life that's too much worrying. That degree of worrying is different for person to person.

So in conclusion what everyone should strive to get rid of is excess unnecessary worry. But it's important to bear in mind that how hard you may try you will never be able to be free from worries hundred percent. After all everyone is human, no one is perfect. Thus the aim is to try and eliminate worries as much as you're able to in order to lead to mentally healthy and happy life. Worrying whether you'll be able to get rid of all those worries inside your head is not a great way to approach the situation. So stop worrying and start working on giving up your worries.

Conclusion

Thank you again for choosing this book!

I hope this book was able to help you to find solutions on how to live without worry.

The next step is to pick the solution that works for you.

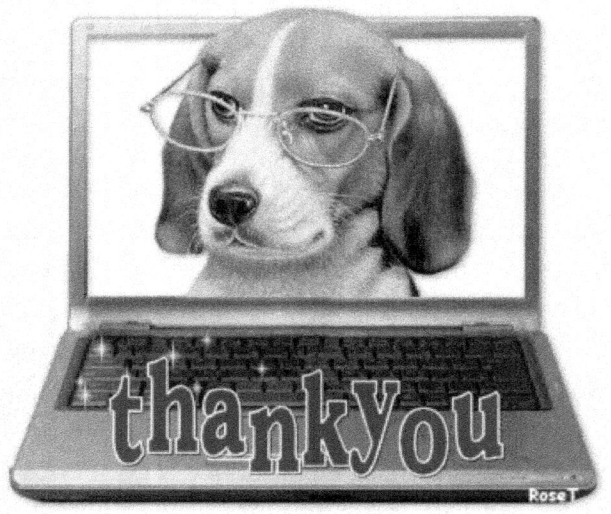

Finally, if you enjoyed this book would you be kind enough to leave a review for this book on Amazon? It'd be greatly appreciated!

Thank you and good luck!

Preview Of 'COPING WITH ANXIETY DISORDER: How to stop Anxiety Tension'

Chapter 1

WHAT IS ANXIETY DISORDER?

Among various human emotions, anxiety is one of the most common emotions. It is an emotional or physical turmoil, which can arise from an event or thoughts. Every person in his or her life experiences anxiety or nervousness in many occasions. Our modern life is full of problems, frustrations, time limits and demands. Arguably, stress is not always bad. A person needs anxiety to some extent; it is required for creativity, learning new things and your survival skills. It helps you to be focused, energetic and prepared. However, when it crosses one's limitation to take stress or it continues for a long period, then it interrupts body's healthy state; it imbalances your body's state of equilibrium.

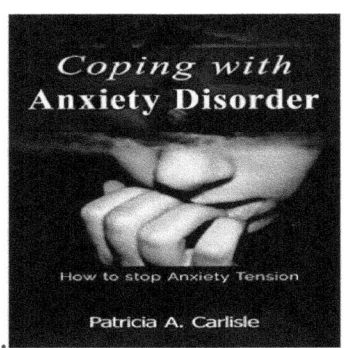

check out the rest of (Coping with Anxiety Disorder: How to stop Anxiety Tension.) on Amazon.

Check Out My Other Books

Below you'll find some of my other popular books that are popular on Amazon and Kindle as well. Alternatively, you can visit my author page on Amazon to see other work done by me.

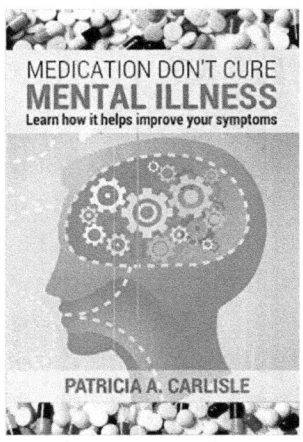

MEDICATION DON'T CURE MENTAL: Learn how it helps improve you symptoms.

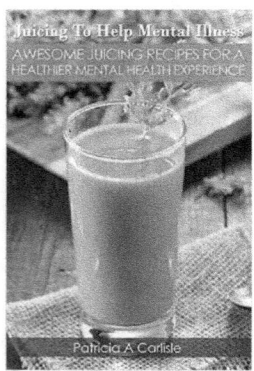

JUICING TO HELP MENTAL ILLNESS: Awesome juicing recipes for a healthier mental health.

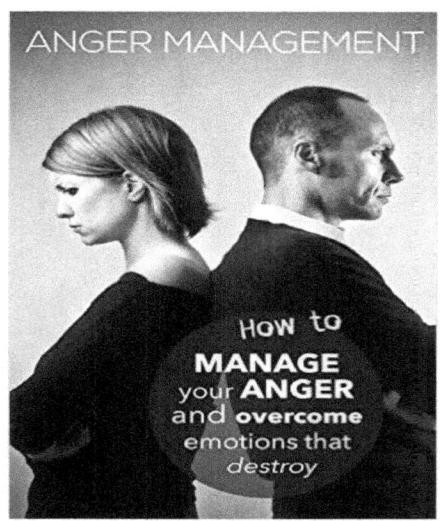

Anger Management: How to manage your anger and overcome emotions that destroy.

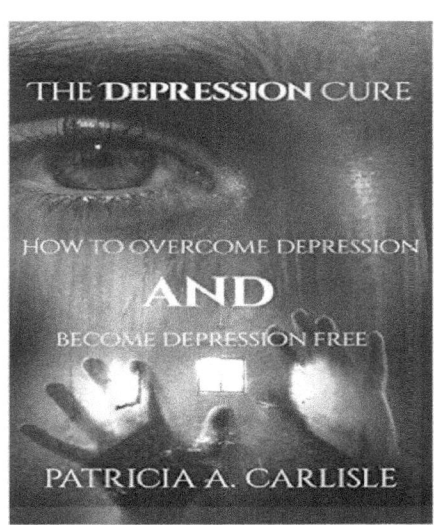

.THE DEPRESSION CURE: How to overcome depression and become depression free.

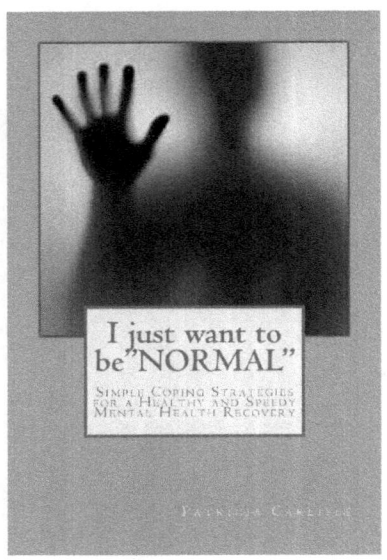

I JUST WANT TO BE "NORMAL" Simple Coping
Strategies for a Healthy and Speedy Mental Health
recovery.

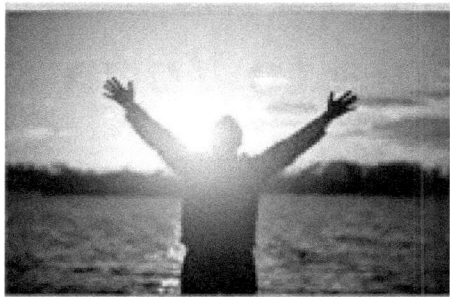

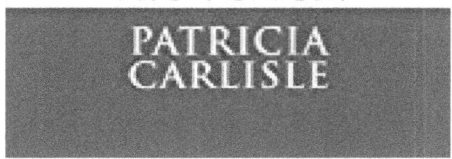

OVER 600 POSITIVE AFFIRMATIONS THAT WILL CHANGE YOUR LIFE: EXPERIENCE THE POWER!

BONUS: SUBSCRIBE TO THE FREE BOOK

Beginners Guide to Yoga & Meditation

"Stressed out? Do You Feel Like The World Is Crashing Down Around You? Want To Take A Vacation That Will Relax Your Mind, Body And Spirit? Well this Easy To Read Step By Step

E-Book Makes It All Possible!"

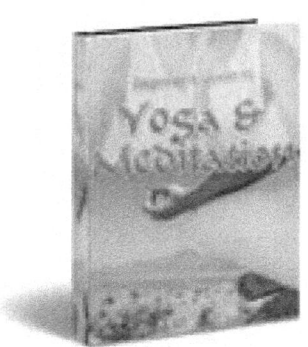

Instructions on how to join our mailing list, and receive a free copy of "Yoga and Meditation" can be found in any of my Kindle eBooks.

NOTES

NOTE

NOTE

NOTES

NOTES

NOTES

NOTES

NOTES

www.ingramcontent.com/pod-product-compliance
Lightning Source LLC
Chambersburg PA
CBHW071019180526
45168CB00003B/1485